Morgan B. Holland/Mullen Press

808 Gleneagles CT #42301

Towson, MD 21218

www.mullenpress.com

contact.us@mullenpress.com

Publisher's Note: We have used our best efforts in preparing the 10-Day Vegan Green Smoothie Cleanse & Detox Book and the information is provided "as is." We make no representation or warranties with respect to the accuracy or completeness of the contents of the book and we specifically disclaim any implied warranties of fitness.

All material in the 10-Day Vegan Green Smoothie Cleanse & Detox Book is provided for your information only and may not be construed as medical advice or instruction. No action or inaction should be taken based solely on the contents of this information; instead, readers should consult appropriate health professionals on any matter relating to their health and well-being.

10-Day Vegan Green Smoothie Cleanse & Detox/ Lamont Connor. -- 1st ed.

ISBN: 978-1-954016-98-9 (paperback)

ISBN: 978-1-954016-97-2 (e-book)

The publisher is not responsible for websites (or their content) that are not owned by the publisher.

Table of
Contents

INTRODUCTION

Welcome to the Vegan 10-Day Green Smoothie Cleanse & Detox!

Congratulations on taking the first step to obtaining and maintaining great health, by feeding your body the nutrients it needs to look good, feel good, have more energy, and be more productive!

Trying to lose excess body fat, unhealthy weight, and eating healthy can be emotionally challenging and frustrating. Many people struggle with losing weight, body fat, health issues, eating habits, obtaining and maintaining a healthy weight and lifestyle. With so many diet fads, fitness regiments, miracle pills and drinks, American's waistlines, heart diseases, and many other avoidable diseases are growing worse yearly. The bottom line is you cannot out train a bad diet, lose weight, and maintain a healthy weight with a poor or temporary diet. It must be a lifestyle change.

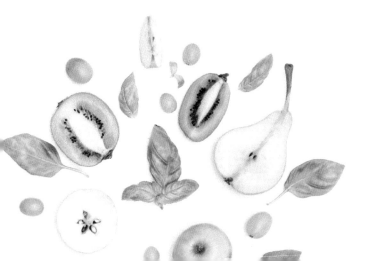

Most people go on a diet temporarily and the weight they lose while on the diet, they gain it back once they come off the diet. People always ask me what is the best diet, I tell them the one that they can maintain for the rest of their life. That is a LIFESTYLE CHANGE. But of course, I believe Whole Food Plant Based Vegan Lifestyle is the best diet. But, I also believe in meeting people where they are at in their journey and improve on that.

A cleanse and a detox is the first step in losing weight. Many people fail to lose weight because they have a lot of build-up toxins and poisons in their gut. But a good cleansing and detox will remove the toxins and poisons from the gut, aid in the weight loss process, and lead to greater health.

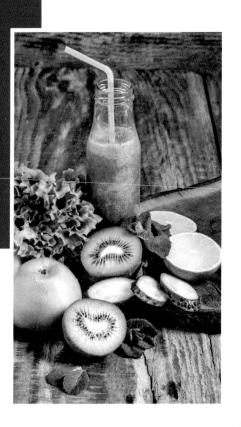

Why I Designed the Vegan 10-Day Green Smoothie Cleanse & Detox?

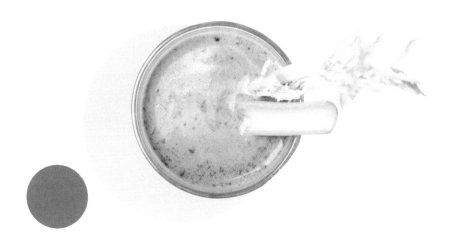

Over a year ago, after years of training myself and others, I suffered a pinched nerve in my neck, which caused lots of pain in my left shoulder. For over a year, to no avail, I tried pain pills, muscle relaxers, cortisone shots, acupuncture, and chiropractor. My final straw was when I got a second epidural and cortisone shot. During the injection, the doctor punctured my lumber, which caused spinal fluid leakage. Spinal fluid leakage causes cerebrospinal fluid that surrounds the brain and spinal cord to leak. Which causes the brain to sag and unbearable headaches when in an upright position. I was confined to bed rest with a pounding headache for 3 weeks and 4 weeks to fully recover. I thank God I was able to fully recover, it takes some people years to recover. As a certified fitness trainer and nutrition consultant, I researched how to use food as medicine. I learned that inflammation in the body is the root cause of most pain, and the main causes of inflammation in the body are excess sugar, meat, animal by-products, dairy, fried, and processed foods. That is when I decided to adopt a Whole Food Plant-Based Vegan Lifestyle. Within a month and a half, the pain in my shoulder was gone. I completed a 5-day smoothie cleanse to transition into the whole food plant-based vegan lifestyle. I lost 8 pounds in 5 days. That's when I decided to design the Vegan 10-Day Green Smoothie Cleanse & Detox. I shared it with some of my clients, family, and friends. Every participant that successfully completed the cleanse lost 10 - 15 pounds in 10 days.

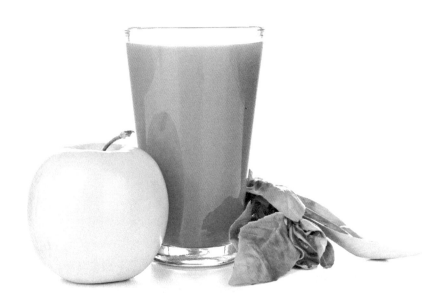

What is the Vegan 10-Day Green Smoothie Cleanse & Detox?

The Vegan10-Day Green Smoothie Cleanse & Detox is 10 smoothies, made up of water, organic green leafy vegetables, organic fresh and frozen fruits, hemp, flax, and chia seeds. If you have diabetes, add a scoop of Plant-Based Vegan Sunwarrior Protein Blend. It provides protein, carbs, and fat. But more importantly, it loaded with essential Minerals & Vitamins.

Nutrient Density

 Mixed Greens: provide calcium, iron, potassium, Vitamin A, C, K, magnesium, folate, fiber, & protein

 Zucchini: provides vitamin C, A, B6, folate, riboflavin, thiamin, magnesium, potassium, manganese, phosphorus, fiber, & protein

 Carrots: provide biotin, potassium, vitamin A, K1, B6, beta carotene, & fiber

 Tomato: provides beta carotene, vitamin A, B, C, E, K, calcium, magnesium, & fiber

Apple: provides vitamin A, C, E, K, B1, B2, B6, potassium, manganese, copper, fiber & protein

Pineapple: provides vitamin A, B6, E, K, calcium, potassium, iron, folate, magnesium, phosphorus, zinc, fiber, & protein

Blueberries: provide vitamin E, B6, C, K1, copper, magnesium, calcium, potassium, phosphorus, iron, zinc, folate, fiber, & protein

Raspberries: provide vitamin A, C, B6, K, E, thiamine, riboflavin, calcium, zinc, potassium, magnesium, copper, iron, fiber, & protein

Strawberries: provide vitamin A, C, B6, K, E, thiamine, riboflavin, calcium, zinc, potassium, magnesium, copper, iron, fiber, & protein

Peaches: provide vitamin A, C, E, K, niacin, folate, iron, choline, potassium, magnesium, phosphorus, manganese, zinc, copper, fiber, & protein

Banana: provides vitamin, C, B6, potassium, magnesium, manganese, copper, fiber, & protein

Orange: provides vitamin C, thiamine, folate, potassium, fiber, & protein

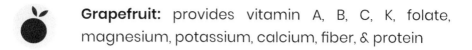

Grapefruit: provides vitamin A, B, C, K, folate, magnesium, potassium, calcium, fiber, & protein

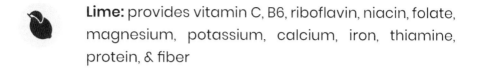

Lime: provides vitamin C, B6, riboflavin, niacin, folate, magnesium, potassium, calcium, iron, thiamine, protein, & fiber

Lemon: provides vitamin C, B1, B2, B5, B6, potassium, calcium, magnesium, iron, copper, manganese, protein, & fiber

Sweet Potato: provides vitamin C, B6, B5, E, A, potassium, magnesium, manganese, fiber, iron, & calcium

Mixed Nuts: provide iron, calcium, potassium, fiber, fat, & protein

Flaxseed: provides potassium, iron, calcium, fiber, fat, & protein

Hempseed: provides manganese, magnesium, phosphorus, folate, vitamin B6, riboflavin, thiamin, potassium, iron, calcium, protein, fat, & fiber

Chia seeds: provide potassium, iron, calcium, protein, fiber, & fat

The Vegan Green Smoothie Cleanse & Detox will

- Help you lose up to 15 lbs. in 10 days.

- Improve gut health.

- Reduce inches around your midsection.

- Increase your energy.

- Clear your mind.

- Detox and remove your craving for sugary, fried, processed, diary, and meat foods.

- Reduce bloating.

- Improve your digestion.

Why Cleanse &
Detox the Body?

An unhealthy gut weakens the immune system and puts the body at risk of sickness, diseases and viruses. Processed foods, excess sugar, dairy, meat and animal by-products lead to an unhealthy gut. Undigested poop in the gut, leads to bad bacteria and overgrown yeast, which makes the immune system weak. Most people have 10 - 25 pounds of undigested poop in their gut. We should periodically detox and cleanse the gut because it's the center of our immune system. After the detox and cleanse, it is important to limit or eliminate processed food, dairy, excess sugar, meat, and animal by-products to help keep the gut healthy and selfheal the body.

How to complete the
Cleanse and Detox

- First thing in the morning make and drink a yogi detox tea on an empty stomach

- In the morning prepare your smoothies for breakfast lunch and dinner

- Between smoothies drink green tea, snack on 1/2 cup of nuts and a fruit, or raw veggie to prevent hunger. (only add fresh squeezed lemon to your tea)

- Stay hydrated, drink 72 oz of water throughout the day, it will help flesh out the toxins

- After the cleansing/detox is completed, take 3 days to slowly reintroduce whole meals into your body. For 2 days drink a green smoothie for breakfast and dinner and eat a light meal (salad) for lunch. Day 3, drink green smoothie for breakfast and eat a light meal for lunch and dinner.

- Drinking a green smoothie every day for 1 or 2 meals is an excellent way to continue to lose weight and or maintain a healthy weight, and to get your daily needed vegetable servings.

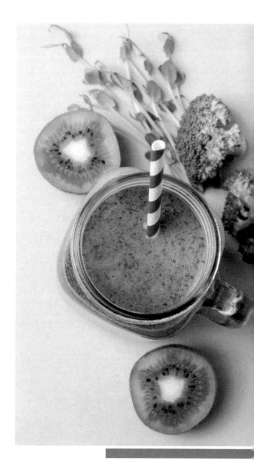

Adjust to fit your schedule

6:00am: Drink 24 oz water and prepare Smoothie.

7:00am: Drink 6-8 oz Yogi Detox Tea

10:00am: Breakfast Smoothie

11:30pm: Drink 24 oz water

12:00pm: (snack) Eat a grapefruit & ½ cup of unsalted mixed nuts.

2:00pm: Lunch Smoothie

3:30pm: Drink 24 oz water

4:00pm: (snack) Eat an apple & ½ cup of unsalted mixed nuts.

6:00pm: Dinner Smoothie

7:30pm: Drink Herbal Green Tea

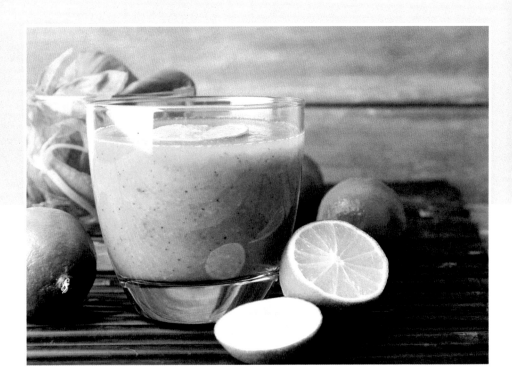

How to Prepare
the Smoothie?

- Each morning, prepare a different smoothie for the day.
- Add and blend the greens and 2-3 cups of water in the blender.
- Then add and blend the fruits and seeds.
- You will end up with about 36 - 48 oz of smoothie.
- Divide them into 3 bottles of 12 - 16 oz of smoothies.
- Place the smoothies in the refrigerator for breakfast, lunch, and dinner. *Purchase 5 days worth.

Market List (buy organic fruits and vegetables) *Purchase 5 days' worth.

For day 1 - 5 days

- 11 ounces of mixed greens
- 11 oz of kale or spinach
- three apples
- 4 pounds of frozen blueberries
- 4 pounds of frozen mixed berries
- 4 pounds of frozen peaches
- 16 oz of flax seeds
- 16 oz of hemp seeds
- 6 ounce of chia seeds
- 2 bananas
- 3 zucchinis

- 3 oranges
- 3 granny apples
- 4 pounds of frozen strawberries
- 3 limes
- Snacks (34 oz unsalted mixed nuts, 5 grapefruits, 5 bananas, sweet potato, raw veggies)
- 5 lemons, box of green herbal tea, Yogi Detox Tea)
- Plant-Based Vegan Sunwarrior Protein Blend

For Day 6 - 10

- 11 oz of mixed greens
- 11 oz of kale or spinach
- 2 granny apples
- 1 lime
- 1 Zucchini
- 4 bananas
- Tomato
- small bag of baby carrots
- 2 lb. of green grapes
- Red apples
- Organic Nut Butter with no added sugar
- Snacks (34 oz unsalted mixed nuts, 5 grapefruits, 5 bananas, sweet potato, raw veggies)
- 5 lemons, box of green herbal tea, Yogi Detox Tea)

DAY 1: Berries Peach Spinach Vegan Smoothie

- 2 handfuls of spinach
- 2 handfuls of mixed greens
- 2 cups of water
- 1 red apple
- 1.5 cups frozen mixed berries
- 1.5 cup of frozen peaches
- 2 tablespoons of flax seeds
- 1 scoop Plant-Based Vegan Sunwarrior Protein Blend (if you have diabetes)

DAY 2: Greens Apple Peach Berries Vegan Smoothie

- 2 handful of spinach
- 2 handful of mixed greens
- 2 cups of water
- 3 tablespoons of chia seeds
- ½ zucchini
- 1 apple
- 1 cup of Frozen mixed berries
- 1 cup frozen peaches
- 1 scoop Plant-Based Vegan Sunwarrior Protein Blend (if you have diabetes)

DAY 3: Green Orange Mixed Berries Vegan Smoothie

- 2 handful of spinach
- 2 handful of mixed greens
- 2 cups of water
- 2 oranges
- 1.5 cup of frozen mixed berries
- 2 tablespoons of flaxseed
- 1 scoop Plant-Based Vegan Sunwarrior Protein Blend (if you have diabetes)

DAY 4: Green Apple Orange Strawberry Vegan Smoothie

- 2 handfuls of mixed greens
- 2 handfuls of spinach
- 3 cups of water
- 1 cup of frozen strawberries
- 1 red apple
- 1 orange
- ½ squeeze lime
- 3 tablespoon hemp seed
- 1 scoop Plant-Based Vegan Sunwarrior Protein Blend (if you have diabetes)

DAY 5: Green Apple Banana Berries Vegan Smoothie

- 2 handful of spinach
- 2 handful of mixed greens
- 3 cups of water
- 1 cup of frozen strawberries
- 1 granny apple
- 1 banana
- 3 tabiespoon chia seed
- 1 scoop Plant-Based Vegan Sunwarrior Protein Blend (if you have diabetes)

DAY 6: Green Lime Apple Berries Vegan Smoothie

- 2 handfuls of spinach
- 2 handful of mixed greens
- 2 cups of water
- 1 granny apples
- 1 cup of frozen strawberries
- 1 cup of frozen blueberries
- ½ squeezed lime
- 1/2 zucchini
- 3 tbsp of chia seed
- 1 scoop Plant-Based Vegan Sunwarrior Protein Blend (if you have diabetes)

DAY 7: Green Banana Nut Butter Vegan Smoothie

- 2 handfuls of kale
- 2 handfuls of mixed greens
- 3 cups of water
- 2 Bananas
- 1 spoonful nut butter
- 2 Tbsp flax seed
- 1 scoop Plant-Based Vegan Sunwarrior Protein Blend (if you have diabetes)

DAY 8: Green Strawberry Banana Vegan Smoothie

- 3 handful and for kale
- 2 cups of water
- 1 banana
- 1 cup of frozen strawberries
- 1 small tomato
- and full of small carrots
- handful of green grapes
- 2 teaspoons of flaxseed

DAY 9: Peach Berry Spinach Vegan Smoothie

- 3 handfuls of spinach
- 2 cups of water
- 1 cup of frozen peaches
- 1 handful of grapes
- 1.5 cup of frozen blueberries
- 3 tablespoons in hemp seed
- 1 scoop Plant-Based Vegan Sunwarrior Protein Blend (if you have diabetes)

DAY 10: Green Apple Berries Vegan Smoothie

- 4 handfuls of mixed greens
- 2 cups of water
- 1 red apple
- 2 cups of frozen mixed berries
- 3 tablespoons and hemp seed
- 1 scoop Plant-Based Vegan Sunwarrior Protein Blend (if you have diabetes)

BONUS SMOOTHIES

Vegan Green Dark Cocoa Banana Smoothie

- 2 handfuls of spinach
- 1 handful of mixed greens
- 2 cups of water
- 1 banana
- 1.5 cup frozen blueberries
- 4 tbsp of 100% cocoa
- 1 handful of dates
- 2 tablespoons of flax seeds
- 1 scoop Plant-Based Vegan Sunwarrior Protein Blend (if you have diabetes)

Green Banana Berries Vegan Smoothie

- 4 handfuls in mixed greens
- 2 cups of water
- 1 banana
- 1.5 cups frozen mixed berries
- 1 Granny Apple
- 2 tablespoons flaxseed
- 1 scoop Plant-Based Vegan Sunwarrior Protein Blend (if you have diabetes)

Green Lime Banana Berry Vegan Smoothie

- 3 handfuls of mixed greens
- 2 cups of water
- 1/2 zucchini
- 2 cups of frozen mixed berries
- 1 banana
- ½ squeezed lime
- 3 tbsp chia seed
- 1 scoop Plant-Based Vegan Sunwarrior Protein Blend (if you have diabetes)

Green Avocado Banana Berry Vegan Smoothie

- 3 handful of mixed greens
- 2 cups of water
- 1 banana
- 1.5 cups of frozen mixed berries
- 1 apple
- 1/2 avocado
- ½ squeeze lime
- 2 tablespoons of flaxseed
- 1 scoop Plant-Based Vegan Sunwarrior Protein Blend (if you have diabetes)

Green Pineapple Banana Berry Vegan Smoothie

- 4 handfuls of mixed greens
- 2 cups of water
- 1 cup of Frozen pineapple
- 1.5 cup of frozen blueberries
- 1 banana
- 1 Tbsp hemp seed
- 1 scoop Plant-Based Vegan Sunwarrior Protein Blend (if you have diabetes)

*The blender you use makes a big difference. Please use a good quality blender, such as a Vitamix or Ninja.

CONCLUSION

The Vegan 10-Day Green Smoothie Cleanse & Detox will accelerate your weight loss, clean your gut, give you more energy, and improve your overall health. It is also an excellent tool to help transition into a whole food plant-based vegan lifestyle.

Made up of nutrient pack leafy greens, fruits, and seeds; the smoothies are tasteful, health, and fulfilling. Your body, mind, and gut will thank you. If you stick with it, this cleansing and detox experience will have a profound effect on your life.

This book provides a shopping list, over 15 green smoothies cleansing & detox recipes, and tips on how to continue to lose weight.

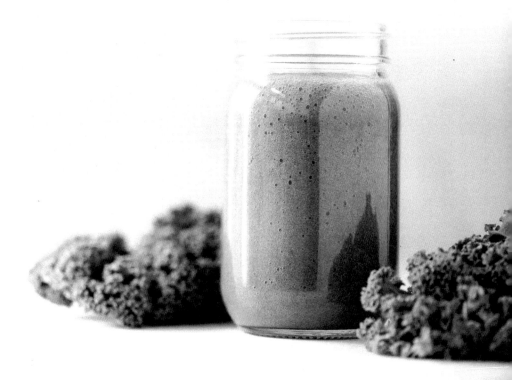

If you successfully complete the Vegan 10-Day Green Smoothie Cleanse & Detox:

- you will lose 10 - 15 lb. in 10 days
- lose belly fat & Inches
- improve gut health
- improve your digestion
- feel better
- look better
- have more energy
- be more productive
- reset your taste buds
- crave healthy food
- detox and eliminate cravings for sugary, dairy, meat, fried and processed foods

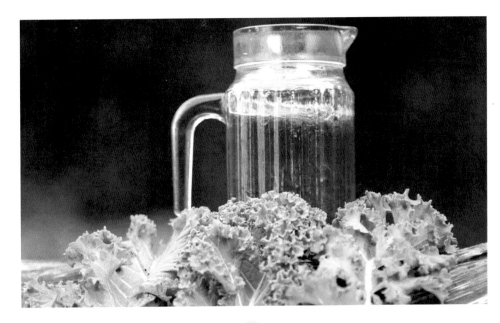

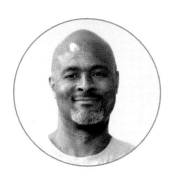

About the
Author

Born and raised in Baltimore, MD as 1 of 17 children, Lamont went on to earn a B.A. in Business Administration from Bowie State University in Bowie, MD and a M.A. in Public Administration from Sojourner Douglas College in Baltimore, MD. He is a husband and father who enjoys spending time with family and friends.

Lamont Connor is the author of 10 Day Vegan Smoothie Cleanse & Detox and owner of Lamont's Fitness Studio. He is a former college football player at Bowie State University, certified fitness trainer, and nutritionist. Lamont Connor helps his clients look better, feel better, have more energy, and become more productive. He provides lifestyle solutions to the strengthening of one's immune system, weight loss, prevent and reverse obesity, and health issues, such as diabetes, high blood pressure, etc.

Lamont is a devoted Christian and Whole Food Plant Based Vegan. He has dedicated his life to healthy living and eating. His passion is to coach, train, educate, and share with others how to use plant based foods and exercising to heal and prevent diseases and viruses, lose unhealthy weight, body fat, stay slim, restore health, look, and feel better. Lamont studied and learned from many great teachers, and is still learning. He has received several certifications including: a fitness trainer and nutrition consultant certification from American Aerobic Sports Medicine Association (AAAI/ISMA), and a nutrition certification from Precision Nutrition. To learn more about products and services Lamont offers visit www.lamontfitness.com.

Made in the USA
Monee, IL
22 November 2021